DELTA-HUMAN SYSTEM

"Better Than Just Going Organic"

A Guide to Principled Eating

By Marcel Ostrow
Certified Sports Nutritionist

Disclaimer:

The information contained in this book is not intended to substitute for medical advice. Any attempt to diagnose or treat an illness should be done under the direction of a healthcare professional. The publisher and author are not responsible for any adverse effects or consequences resulting from the use of the suggestions, procedures or preparations discussed in this book. If the reader has any questions, it is strongly recommended they consult their health care professional.

ISBN-13:
978-1460904282

ISBN-10:
1460904281

Armed with a proper knowledge about food...
...Ultra-health-conscious-citizens

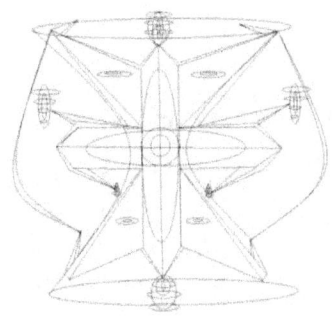

It is time...
... To become a Delta-human

TABLE OF CONTENTS

INTRODUCTION
Better Than Just Going Organic

In times like these, we need to keep it straight and simple. We need a system that will protect a person from the inside-out. We need more information about ourselves and how we should eat. It is more than simply picking organic over conventional because there is much more to human nutrition than just worrying about the quality and origin of our foods. By first addressing the importance of our own knowledge in regards to basic human needs, we begin to take the steps necessary to shield ourselves, and our loved ones, from the food disasters that are happening all around us. The Center for Disease Control and Prevention (CDC) predicted that this generation of children would be the first in our nation's history not to live as long as their parents. America and the world need better food quality, but more than anything, we need to learn how and what to eat.

Producers in a free market society make a profit by fulfilling consumer's demands, however; if we have our own long-term benefit as a top priority, we must begin demanding only quality *real food*. The change starts with each individual. We must create a demand for only the best foods for human nutrition. Right here and now, you have the power to achieve your goals by changing many things in your life, and food is one of the most important.

This book will help you rediscover just how much you can actually do to help yourself achieve success with food. The Delta-human System will give you tools, realistic examples, contrasts, evidence, and reasons to empower you to take control of your own body by raising a strong awareness about your basic human nature and about the advantages that come with having a well-nourished body.

Principled Eating

Principled eating is the habitual practice of eating according to the principles given in the Delta-human System. *Principled eating* can improve your life drastically by simplifying your meals. It works because it brings together and clarifies, many of the over-looked factors about food and human digestion. You will be given key concepts to strengthen your food selection mechanism. With the Delta-human System way to *principled eating*, you can take advantage of simple home meals that can help boost your productivity. Imagine taking just 5-10 minutes to prepare a meal that will nourish your body and mind by making you feel great, instead of wasting your resources in complicated recipes and cooking procedures that might taste good, yet actually do you more harm than good. You can win with food every day simply by taking the time to understand how to maximize the efficiency of your nutrient absorption with the principles in this book. The Delta-human System is your guide to a more efficient change. Re-read it as many times as is necessary to understand the basic concepts. Be prepared to experience, within reason, the changes you have probably wanted all your life regarding your health and appearance. The Delta-human System simplifies the process of food selection for you. This guide addresses the most important issues for busy city people that must make the best out of the foods they have available.

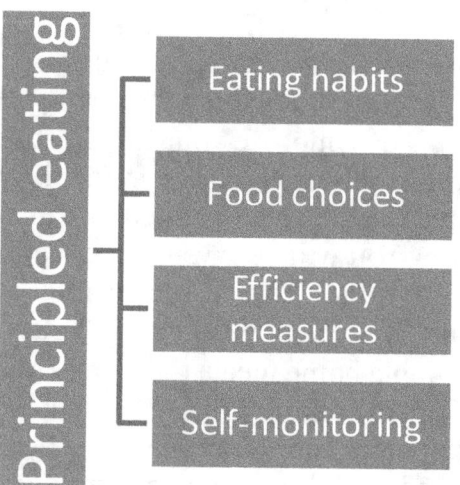

Principled eating is a courageous attempt to remain in harmony to what nature intended for you. The pages to come will explain just what these principles are and how to apply them with the Delta-human System.

WHAT IS THE DELTA-HUMAN SYSTEM?

The Delta-human System is the alternative to supplements, chemicals or everything else that has failed; the one fully workable system that stimulates and empowers you to get the correct foods that your body needs to achieve its full mental and physical potential. A Delta-human only consumes food for its true purpose: to produce the energy required to survive. It is the art of eating to live while avoiding toxicity. You will learn to protect your body and mind from harmful illusions and fake foods that abusive marketing tactics, culture, and other forces, have trained you to mindlessly allow into your life. You can increase productivity and add years of health to your life with the principles in this book.

To begin with the Delta-human System, we will create a new name for you. You will no longer be a "regular" human, per se; one that simply reacts to his environment. You will create a new standard, a new identity that will make it easier to make the change you seek. You will become a Delta-human; a more principled human. A Delta-human is any individual who has mastered (often heroically) his basic physical needs. One who has identified all the factors needed to sustain his optimal self under any circumstance. Whether he chooses to grow his own food in a farm or to buy the food he needs in the vast supplies of a modern city market, he can implement either one successfully with the proper mindset.

A Delta-human has a wealth of energy, walks with a bounce, moves with skill, precision, and makes lightning fast decisions that boost his survival despite all the negative advertising or cultural influences in his immediate surroundings. A Delta-human can drastically improve the life of those around him. Friends and family are often amazed and captivated by the discipline and often rare habits of the Delta-human. The Delta-human gains respect and admiration when people notice the health, beauty and energy that radiates from their bodies. A wind of curiosity surrounds them. With the Delta-human System, you inherit a new world of choices. You also acquire the power to choose to help those around you suffering from poor eating habits (the vast majority). It is perfectly valid to care for those you love, but get the system working for you before you try it with others. Speak success from your own success and not from memorized repetition.

With the Delta System, you will recognize a world hidden from plain view. You will discover powerful secrets of nutrition. You will bring out your true power.

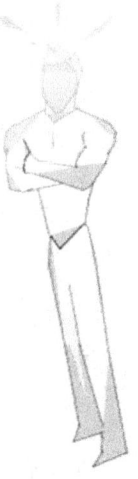

This system is not based on chemicals or miracle potions like most other programs out there. The Delta-human System is a new and "hands-on" type of knowledge that allows you to take full control of your body in ways never before attempted. You can achieve the body of your dreams as well as the energy and knowledge required to maintain it through simple, yet powerful identification techniques based on historical human nature, common sense, and doing what feels right for your body.

With the Delta-human System, you can realize many benefits including:

- Health and longevity

- Naturally smooth and beautiful skin (no more pimples or dryness)

- Increased vigor and energy

- Flawless digestion (prevent ulcers, gastritis, colitis, gases or bloating)

- Reduce waist size quickly and naturally

- Advantages that can make a lasting change in you and your family

The Delta-Human System is simple and basic, however, it must be properly understood and its rules implemented within every decision and food choice. It is a system to guide your habits. Making the Delta-human System effective, requires discipline and constant thought. You may apply the concepts to your own life immediately to start realizing these benefits. The Delta System is with you, protecting you at home, in restaurants, and at supermarkets. For best results, you should re-read the system immediately a 2nd time after the first, and at least once per month from there on to keep your mind on track.

Only a habit can get rid of another habit, and the best habits will be easier to implement if you know what your basic needs are first. Please interact with other Delta-Humans by visiting Deltahuman.com to enter your own posts in the forums, feed-back contact boxes, facebook, etc. Share your troubles and successes with others like you, who really care about their health.

HOW TO USE THIS GUIDE:

Rule #1: Have the homeostasis octagon (see page 60) in front of you all the time. You may print a blank "fill-in" copy at www.deltahuman.com/tools.html

Rule #2 Understand the principles in the *Sample diets*(in the appendix) and then customize your own.

Rule #3: Be willing to make changes in your life. A certain degree of independent thinking is needed. Also, you must be willing to invest in quality food for yourself. This is a health priority worth the amount you invest multiplied many times over.

Rule #3 Apply the Delta-human System while observing your body. Never forget that what you feel is important. Feeling great comes naturally with the great food choices suggested in this System, but keep track of what works best for you and your unique metabolism. Never remain doing something that hurts.

Rule #4 Stay focused. Figuring out the Delta-human System requires time and concentration. You must look for the appropriate time and place to read this document. The time and concentration you are willing to give will make this system that much more effective in your future life.

Rule #5 You are becoming a Delta-human…It is not easy…be proud, success will come…

IMPORTANT: If you wish to start right away, simply follow the 4 sample diets found in the appendix (pg 70). Begin by alternating diets 1,2 and 3, while keeping an alkaline day (diet 4) 2-3 times per week. After reading this book you may customize your own diets using *principled eating.*

For example: a week with the following diets:

Sun - 4/ Mon – 1/ Tue – 2 / Wed – 4 / Thu – 3 / Fri – 1 / Sat – 2

NOTE TO THE READER: This book is intended as an informational guide, the concepts and techniques described here are meant to supplement dietary habits and not substitute for professional medical care. For treatment of serious ailments, consult a qualified healthcare provider.

POINT 1:

The Basic Misunderstanding...

Few people realize the true meaning of food. The average American has confused its true meaning and with that, has diminished his chances of achieving optimal performance in his or her life. The only valid meaning for food is energy. The energy in food comes in many forms, be it proteins, fats, naturally occurring sugars, fibers, vitamins, minerals, etc. Today, however; food is equated with enjoyment. We as human beings have developed sensitive flavor receptors in the tongue that allowed us to naturally enjoy the act of eating. This was our natural and evolutionary advantage for millions of years in the search for food in the wild since the days we were wandering nomads. With flavorful delight, we gave preference to sweet things like fruits, enjoyed savory meat and were motivated to tolerate the pain of capturing a honey comb. We also, instinctively, rejected dangerous foods because of their bitter or unpleasant taste. The bottom line regarding food is primarily <u>eating it to survive</u>, and only as a secondary consequence, to enjoy it. Enjoyment alone must never be the main reason for selecting food. Today, the act of internalizing this fact is more important than ever because our own taste buds work against us in a highly commercial and completely impulsive society like America. Today, a person ignoring sound nutrition principles and eating only to enjoy food is almost inevitably heading toward physical and mental disaster. He or she will innately gravitate around the sweetest and saltiest foods on the market, in other words, this person will use garbage as the fuel his body requires to survive. How do you think this person looks and feels? This is why you as a Delta-human must adhere to *principled eating* and not follow bodily impulses without thought.

So be it, that we will choose food that is healthy and not necessarily the tastiest while applying this system. Mastering this habit is an acquired Delta-human advantage.

NEW CONCEPT: Pervasive Homeostasis

This symbol: $\overline{\triangle}$ stands for the word homeostasis. It is a Delta symbol or triangle, the most stable of all shapes which stands for *balance*. It has a crescent on top which symbolizes *pervasiveness*; the homeostasis symbol represents the perfect and ideal state for your body <u>to be</u> in both, time and space. When a stable homeostasis is attained, you have become a *Delta-human*, you have mastered your body's physical and mental requirements for sustained well-being. **This is the goal of the Delta-human System.** Homeostasis is only achieved through the combined efforts of your mind and body in procuring energy through *principled eating*. Refer to the *Homeostasis octagon* in the conclusion (pg. 60) to see what factors must be controlled and aligned within your environment to achieve *Pervasive homeostasis*.

POINT 2:

PROCUREMENT OF REAL FOODS:

One of the first diets to make a significant impact in modern man's notion of food was the *Atkins diet*. This diet made specific breakthroughs regarding the way we digest protein and its many positive effects to human health, especially weight-loss. Then we had the *Metabolic typing diet* revolution which assures us that we are all different and need different types of foods, yet there is something that remains constant, and that is that the synthetic pseudo-foods most of us are buying today are not nature-intended for any human being regardless of his or her metabolic type.

Today a new type of diet comes to our attention: the controversial Paleolithic diet, better known as P*aleo-diet*. We are challenged to rethink our eating habits and contrast them with those of our ancestors; to assess natural foods versus man-made foods. This realization is making health-conscious

13

people look at sustainable and organic practices no longer as an inefficient burden to our economy, but as a basic human need that we all depend on for optimal health. The road toward getting back the food as nature intended for us should become a priority once people realize that nature equates to justice; a system of balances that can never be cheated. Behind our concrete walls and computerized lives, is our delicate human nature which we should fully embrace with our minds and bodies in all ways possible.

Only real food is properly metabolized by the human body without toxic or adverse effects. Taking a look at human evolutionary studies is strongly encouraged for anyone with a genuine interest in human nutrition. You can find out a lot of information on evolutionary diets in books and over the internet. These diets are pioneers in the identification of *real foods*. In simple terms, evolutionary diets point out that you should strive to eat only natural foods. Foods that you would be able to pluck out from the ground such as carrots, broccoli and cress, or that you would pull down from trees such as cherries and coconuts. Very important are nutritious animal proteins like eggs, meat, fish, etc. These are real foods that our human make-up has been accustomed to for millions of years, much before discovering the act of cooking. Within the discoveries of the *Paleo-diet*, we find important factual conclusions that lead us to see bulk foods such as grains, beans and potatoes as alien to the original human diet, and that furthermore, may even be responsible for troubled digestion or other problems in which individual tolerance to these foods may vary. If you are not familiar with it already, go right now and read about the *Paleo-diet* by visiting the following website: http://paleolithicdiet.wordpress.com/2008/06/22/original-introduction/.

Procuring only real foods may be hard at times. Many communities have local farmer's markets where it is possible to get the freshest seasonally grown food. People with no access to local food, however; should keep in mind that conventional food markets are fine if we are careful to select the food. To be able to select the highest quality "packaged" food, if need be, you should identify questionable ingredients in food. *Wholefoods Market*, is one of the largest influences of the organic movement in America today. Their presence alone is a wake-up call for many health-conscious Americans. Their website contains a useful list of "unacceptable ingredients in food", which you may print from the following url: http://www.wholefoodsmarket.com/products/unacceptable-ingredients.php . Always read your food labels while remembering to also discard anything containing sugar. (All types of sugar, including high-fructose syrups, white or even brown sugar).

Briefly stated, you should strive to ingest mostly *organic* fruits, vegetables, and proteins. This is done to avoid unnatural added byproducts of all-for-profit modern day agri-business attempts to cheat nature. Namely, things like growth hormones, nitrates, preservatives, dioxins, pesticides, herbicides, and other chemicals that can bio-accumulate in the cells of your body and cause toxic responses and other abnormalities.

Note: The Paleo diet's discoveries are highly supported by the Delta System; however, the Delta System holds the following views regarding dairy, salt, nuts, and oatmeal (a grain). It also includes a warning about fish, meat, and oils.

On dairy: While the Paleo-diet regards all dairy, besides mother's milk, as not suited for human consumption, the Delta System suggests that this is true only for all processed (homogenized, pasteurized and hormone added) dairy products. There are real life examples of people living to incredibly old age while consuming fresh (usually raw) dairy in moderate amounts. Such an example is found in the tea with butter that the Hunza people of Eastern Pakistan (who often live to be 120) so eagerly enjoy.

Their cows and goats produce milk richer in ADA and ARA; this is milk of the highest order because they are fed grass, and not just any grass, but one that has been irrigated with mineral rich glacial waters. In America however, it is almost impossible to get fresh unprocessed milk because of tough FDA regulations and other sanitary measures. After all, there are valid safety concerns with the handling of milk and in guaranteeing that it is not contaminated. For many people, it makes sense to reduce or simply avoid dairy for that reason. People that are prone to having congested nasal passages should observe if the removal of dairy, particularly sharp and over-processed cheeses might help to clear-up the throught and respiratory tracks. Dairy is not recommended by the Delta-human System unless it is of a very high nature.

On Salt: While the Paleo diet advocates an abstinence of salt, The Delta System openly endorses its use on the grounds of empirical observations. Just ask your local vet what happens to a cow without a salt block. Or what happens to a human being with hyponatremia. Salt is necessary for all living beings in a moderate amount. You lose salt when you perspire, sweat, excrete mucous and tears. You must, eventually, replace it. The reason is electrical. Your body has an electrical circuitry of nerve impulses. Sodium and potassium are the negative/positive ions in your cells. When you have an imbalance of sodium/potassium ratios, you can feel tired, dizzy, or like you are going to pass out. This condition is called hyponatremia. Conventional table salt, however, is not recommended for many reasons. The only salts endorsed by this System for their outstanding purity, trace element content and properties are: Sea, Himalayan, and Celtic salts.

How much sodium per day is it ok to ingest? According to the American Heart Association: less than one tea-spoon (2,400mg) per day. It takes about ¼ of a tea-spoon to balance daily sodium requirements. This does not imply that you must have salt every day. This should just give you an idea on how to measure salt consumption. Do not go over the limits, but do not neglect much needed sodium from your diet either. Will salt alter the blood pressure? It may or may not, depending on the individual's physical make-up. People with high blood pressure problems must consult with their doctors before taking salt because only a doctor can determine if there are other complications involved.

On oatmeal: Oatmeal is the grain that the Delta-human recommends most out of all other grains. There is still not a high degree of certainty on the issue of grains; however, the *Paleo-diet* is against the consumption of all grains. Oatmeal is the exception in the Delta-human System for a couple of reasons. The first reason is empirical: old fashioned oatmeal has been part of the diet of many long-lived Americans. It is lower than wheat, corn and rice on the glycemic index, which makes it a steadier source of energy. It is also less likely to spike your blood/sugar levels and give you a sugar crash. Oats have twice as much protein as wheat and corn. Rolled oats can even be eaten raw, although they are easier to digest when cooked. It is a hearty food that is locally available for all Americans at a relatively low cost. And the favorite reason is because they constitute a hearty source of bulk calories that is loaded with energy. The taste is also very pleasant, just adding a dash of ground cinnamon and a bit of sea salt makes it very delicious. Like all grains however, oats can cause acidity in the body if taken every day as we will discuss in point 6,thus having oatmeal for breakfast is recommended no more than 3-4 times per week. Brown rice, sprouted wheat (as in sprouted breads), and barley are the next better grain choices, although people with gluten sensitivity should be cautious. Low grain diets are best.

On Nuts: Nuts must be eaten as fresh as possible. Their natural oils many times go rancid and the consumer seldom notices. This is why it is preferable to get nuts in their shell and crack them open while they are still fresh. Nuts should be eaten in small amounts because they are very highly packed with slow-digesting fat and do not mix well with other foods.

The ideal ratio of omega-6 to omega-3 in humans is 4:1. Nuts however, can cause an excess of omega-6 in the body and as a consequence, deplete omega-3. Walnuts for instance, are seen as a great source of omega-3, but their ratio to omega-6 is 10:1. So this actually creates a large deficit in the omega-3 which then must to be remedied by eating other omega-3 rich foods. Therefore, when it comes to nuts, eat them alone and complement your diet with omega 3 rich-foods such as fresh flax or chia seeds.

Note that many seeds and nuts are easier to digest after soaking or sprouting them. Almonds for instance, should be soaked to improve their digestibility and nutrition profile. Soaking them also removes harmful enzyme inhibitors and tannic acid. Soak almonds in cool water and if possible drain the soaked water after 20-40 minutes. Then add fresh water and continue soaking for another 8-12 hours. You may continue and sprout them if you like. Being that the almond skin is potentially irritating to the lining of the stomach and intestines, the almonds should be blanched (following the soaking).

To blanch almonds:

Place the soaked almonds in a saucepan of boiling water.
2. Time seven (7) seconds.
3. Remove from heat.

4. Drain and cover almonds with cold water to cool.
5. Press almond between thumb and forefinger to slip off skin.

You can also try blanching them in warm water (15-30 seconds in hot water from the faucet.)

Warning about fish: Avoid fish unless you know it is pristine and safe. Toxicity in our oceans is worse than most of us would expect. Mercury and PCB's can be a real threat to your health. Especially worrisome, is the potential neurological damage from the exposure to these contaminants that tend to bio-accumulate in seafood. Explore the Environmental Defense Fund's website for relevant information:
http://www.edf.org/page.cfm?tagID=1540

On meat, chicken and eggs: Meat is not what it used to be. Stick with "organic-grass-fed beef", and organic-free-range chicken and eggs. Be especially careful with conventional organ meats like liver and kidney, as they are organs that can accumulate many toxins and should therefore have a pristine origin. Meat should be cooked enough to kill bacteria, but never must it be burnt or charred. Doing so will deplete its protein quality and will produce HCA's, the carcinogenic chemicals that are produced from cooking meat at high temperatures. For more information about HCA's visit the following link from the National Cancer Institute: http://www.cancer.gov/cancertopics/factsheet/Risk/heterocyclic-amineshttp://www.edf.org/page.cfm?tagID=15705

On oils: Do not cook with oils, as their chemical composition changes at high temperatures and they lose their beneficial properties and become toxic. Once oils oxidize, they create free radicals that disturb the protective function of antioxidants. We only recommend Coconut oil for cooking as it is more resistant to heat and will not burn like other oils, keeping in mind that only light to medium heat should be used with coconut oil. Olive and flax-seed oils (great for getting essential omega 6 and 3 respectively), are recommended as cold and uncooked salad dressings. The problem with buying oils is that they are very volatile and go rancid much quicker than most people would expect. A couple of things can be done to minimize the problem.
1) Buy oil in small bottles: this way you can use the bottle quickly, once it is open, air starts to oxidize the oils fast, so replace the cap immediately. 2) Keep oils in a dark and cool place. Avoid foods containing hyper-heated oils. Fried foods and snacks such as potato chips many times contain cheap oils that come from cottonseed; since cotton is often sprayed with chlorophenol insecticides, the amount of pesticides and

toxins can be higher in these oils in addition to consuming over-heated oxidized oils and a recently found cancer-promoting substance called acrylamide which is found in most fried foods. Baking, steaming, grilling, and boiling are healthier alternatives for heating foods.

On vitamin/mineral supplements: In order to have ideal health, we need certain nutrients. We know that we need a complex mix of vitamins, minerals, amino-acids, fats, proteins and more of these nutritional categories, but what does this translate into in simpler terms? Should we buy supplements? Research has shown that many times these vitamins and minerals are simply not absorbed by the body in their commercial isolated forms. Time-tested reality can almost assure us that the only natural and true pathway for vitamin and mineral absorption is through good-old-raw-food sources. Multi-vitamin and mineral supplements, however, are indeed recommended for the average city dweller because most people do not have the means or the access, to the rich and raw food that our ancestors ate.

The reason most of us do need extra nutrients, is not only because of the depletion of our farm lands causing nutrient deficient vegetables and fruits; in an ironic way, it is even more obvious than that. Centuries ago, our ancestors the hunter-gatherers, would not wash vegetables or roots. They simply ate them with all the glorious dirt around them. Same applied to their water which would be taken from flowing rivers and lakes. This water had higher concentrations of mineral-rich clay or soil, nothing like the highly filtered water from our pipelines. Many indigenous people around the world have much lower incidences of heart disease, cancers, diabetes, tooth decay, obesity, and other modern day health issues, partly because of the natural mineral clays that they consume. This rich soil possesses many basic minerals and trace elements that our bodies require in very small quantities. The real challenge facing modern man is getting these nutrients from foods alone in a society that cannot tolerate the slightest spec of anything resembling dirt on any of our foods. Besides, even if we did, would we want to eat even the slightest amount of pesticide ridden dirt around our conventional carrots? Despite the awkwardness of the idea of eating dirt, there are well documented cases in which certain natural clays and minerals were used with great effectiveness by ancient societies for the treatment of various illnesses throughout the centuries. This form of natural supplementation will become stronger in the future of natural medicine and a powerful alternative to cure mineral deficiencies. Today, there are sophisticated and relatively inexpensive ways to know your specific mineral excesses or deficiencies. You are encouraged to take a hair chemical analysis and/or a blood chemical analysis with a qualified holistic health-care provider to determine your own unique mineral balances and to detect any harmful levels of heavy metal poisoning. These tests take out the guess work, and tell you what specific mineral supplements can help you meet these mineral requirements and regulate any imbalances.

On Sugar: Let's remember that sugar, the most widely consumed drug today, is not part of the Delta-human diet. Sugar was introduced in Europe in the late 12th century as "sweet salt", and was for many years locked up in apothecary shops and labeled as a dangerous drug, until people started slowly incrementing its consumption to the outrageous levels we consume today. Sugar plays with your sense of taste and stimulates you to buy poor food choices. Moreover, sugar happens to be a preservative that keeps food on the shelf much longer; it is no wonder they put sugar in everything these days (read your labels, even things considered healthy like granola bars, flavored yogurts, or breakfast cereals can all have massive amounts of sugar). Sugar is not well metabolized in your body. Sugar is the purest and most refined form of carbohydrate out there. Sugar has addictive properties that you must learn to fence-off. You must take sugar and its substitutes, such as high-fructose corn syrup, out of your life forever. You must start by recognizing sugar in every food you intake.

Sugar is a primary cause of countless physical, mental and emotional problems. Diets high in sugar are linked to obesity, diabetes, tooth decay, depression, etc. It affects people in different ways depending on their type of metabolism, but it will affect you in the long run and your teeth alone will attest to that. So first and foremost, stay away from sugar, sugary foods and beverages such as desserts or sodas, and stay like that as close to forever as possible. Be strong and bear with yourself because you are up against social convenience for this simple fact. You will understand how hard it is to avoid sugar if you haven't already figured that out. One day, all the people will realize what sugar really does and stop its production, but until that happens, you will have to exert tough thinking and discipline in your food selection in order to avoid it. For those of you, who need a sweet touch, try the natural sugar substitute stevia, but only until your need for sweetness fades with time and discipline. Do not however, abuse sugar substitutes, even natural ones, as they are a false alarm for the brain which by the sweet taste, expects a high caloric load, when in fact, there are no calories in "0-calorie" sweeteners. Only use them sparingly for the purpose of controlling sugar-anxiety and cravings (all dependency symptoms from sugar addiction), while preparing for a sugar-free lifestyle.

How much food should we eat?

For a Delta Human, the most important aspect of food is its nature and quality. After we have procured good quality "real foods" as discussed above, we can then go into the technical aspects of food such as caloric balancing. Not all food is equal; we should not say; "I will get "x" amount of calories from raw carrots and "x" amount from a bowl of ice cream", like most calorie conscious people think. The carrots are a high quality food that should be counted toward our daily calorie needs. The ice cream, on the other hand, is loaded with calories, but the process to metabolize it is different because of the sugary/dairy-heaviness inherent in the mix of ice cream ingredients. Always rely on the quality of the calories, never on just the calories themselves.

Essentially, energy consumed must equal the amount of energy spent. A hypothetical "0" should be our daily maintenance goal. Do we need to look at the caloric content of each and every food? The answer is yes. You must use your most powerful and wondrous tool; your mind. You must use it to know it all about food; the research is readily available for everybody. You just need to be interested and willing to find out.

Using your mind effectively is the secret to achieving your goals in everything in life, including of course, your basic nutritional needs. We must realize that discarding processed and sugary foods from our diets means that we will need to put in their place larger amounts of natural foods. We should understand that a human body will need as many calories as approximately 11 times your body weight in pounds. For example, if your desired weight is 175 lbs., then you would need 175 x 11 = 1925 calories per day just to maintain your basic metabolic processes functioning. Furthermore, if you are an active person that, for instance, runs and works-out for 2 hours in a day and spends 700 calories doing so, then you would have to intake 1925 + 700 = 2625 calories for every day that you do this specific workout.

When it comes to selecting your caloric needs, it is good to keep in mind that the portion size of your meals should seldom exceed the size of your closed fist. Thus many small meals in a day work better for digestive purposes.

QUICKLY CALCULATE YOUR APROXIMATE METABOLIC CALORIC NEEDS USING THE PREVIOUS FORMULA (Your weight in pounds x 11). THEN YOU CAN USE THE FOLLOWING RESOURCES TO GET THE CALORIES IN SPECIFIC FOODS AND THE CALORIES YOU MUST ADD ACCORDING TO YOUR SPECIFIC ACTIVITIES.

☛ External Resources:

To see the calories in specific foods, use the calorie calculator chart at: http://www.deltahuman.com/tools.html

To help you keep track of how many calories you need depending on your SPECIFIC activities, refer to the following website: http://www.healthstatus.com/calculate/cbc

Longevity studies show that *Caloric Restriction* (CR) can increase the lifespan of lab animals (monkeys, rats, and insects). This has been a controversial topic when applied to humans because it is so hard to measure its long-term effects. In response to this information, The Delta-human System concludes that if your diet is made up of *real foods*, then you can reduce your number of determined calories since you are getting quality nutrients from nutrient-dense foods like meat, as opposed to empty calories like the ones from white bread. It is recommended to start-off with your calculated caloric needs and then adjust them down for *caloric restriction* benefits. For example: for a person that needs 2,400 calories, try reducing it to 2,200 derived from high quality foods. Test to see if your body feels better doing so. Always listen to your body. Try *caloric restriction* and adjust your energy intake according to your energy needs and the way your body feels over time.

The most important principle regarding food procurement is this: Do not focus on avoiding bad food, instead, focus on filling your refrigerator and kitchen with *real foods*. In other words, get so many *real food* that there will be no room for the "bad foods" to enter. You can see a recommended food list in the appendix. Be aware that good and bad foods are always competing for a place in your house. Never give way to even a little bad, because the good foods are integral parts of a delicate balance. If you eat something bad, the whole system's steady progress may be interrupted. This is why pristine things are so precious and rare. It takes great effort to develop purity and consistency. Like a premium diamond, Delta-humans shine with the beauty that comes from well-nourished bodies. Many people rebel against real effort done either by themselves or others by using a phrase like: "just live a little", or "in the end, we are all going to die anyways". This is why they fail. It is not that the person following the Delta-human System 100% is "not living" or is "too strict", realize that it is black or white. There are no grays, you are either eating for health or not. Reaching perfection for the sake of perfection is not the point, but striving for perfection to the best of your ability is. Ask yourself whenever you are looking for an excuse to avoid discipline, if you are secretly trying to cheat yourself. Realize how absurd attempting to hide your nature from your own self can be. If you feel that you are being too hard on yourself, then establish where your limits are. Being comfortable within your limits is necessary, but sometimes you just have to push the comfort level to adapt to today's challenges. Remember that nature acts never in haste. Use your knowledge and principles, compare them to your actions, and then forever improve those actions with discipline. This powerful interaction with your physical reality (your resources) and consciousness (your identification of those resources) inevitably unfolds into a wonderful discovery of your inner power.

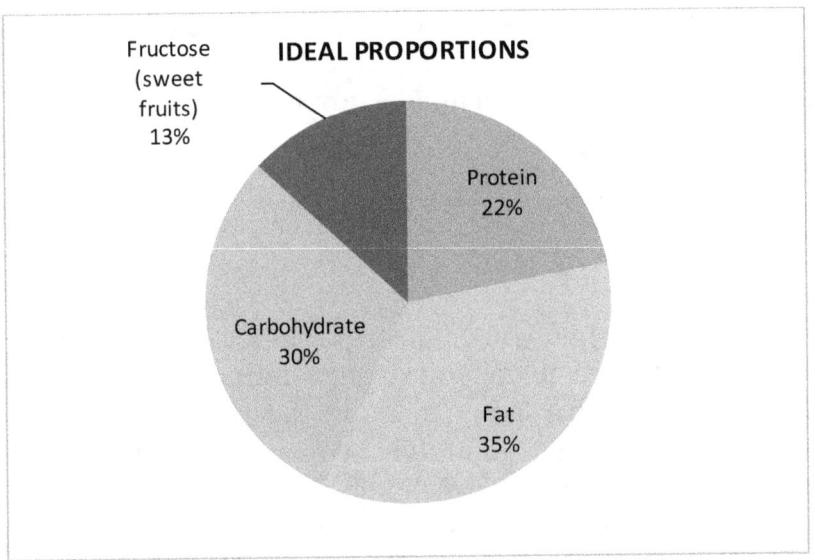

For a diet to be balanced, the Delta-human System recommends that **Protein** (varied and lean) should account for about 22% of your total calories. **Carbohydrates** (predominantly low-glycemic vegetables and greens) should account for about 35%, **Fat** (predominantly monounsaturated and omega-rich fats from vegetable and nut oils along with some pristine animal fat such as the one found in salmon) should account for about 30%, and **Fructose** (fruits) for about 13% of you daily caloric needs. These values are calculated from comparing hunter-gatherer macronutrient ratios (very high in protein and fat and low in carbohydrates) versus the modern American ones (mostly carbohydrate based) in an attempt to balance out the disparities and opting for a middle ground.

NEW CONCEPT: Identification Lock

It is normal that while you get involved in reading this guide, your mind will start giving you strong warnings every time you are near food that should be avoided, sort of like an alarm inside your head. You might be in a store or at a social gathering and have to make a choice. In other words, to be under financial or social pressure to eat low-quality food. But do not panic, this alarm is a normal effect called an **Identification Lock**. An *Identification lock* can be better described as a feeling of panic to avoid something that you know is not good. For example, you are going to buy fish at the supermarket one day and you notice that the bluefish there are very cheap. You want to find out more about the bluefish and you do some online research and found out that there are health alerts for dangerous levels of mercury and PBC's in bluefish. On the other hand, you know that Wild Alaskan Salmon is a bit more expensive, but that it is relatively safer to eat. You act on the knowledge and not the impulse (This might seem like mere common sense, but huge mistakes can go by unnoticed when you do not take your internal warnings seriously. Social pressure and attitudes such as: "but everyone else is buying it", can make you fail at using what should be common sense and cause you to tune-out). An *identification lock* instantly comes to your mind telling you to pay the extra 2 dollars for the Alaskan Salmon than for the cheaper bluefish. You then buy Alaskan salmon without regret because safety comes first.

Here is an example of an *Identification lock* under social pressure: you are at a family reunion in which your aunt made her famous glazed cinnamon rolls. You feel compelled to eat them, the smell of cinnamon-sugar and baked bread makes your mouth water. How can you say no if she is staring right at you with her dessert in hand? The answer is: with honesty. An alarm (*Identification lock*) telling you not to eat this comes to your head like a punch, and you act on it with honesty and gentleness. Your example will help everyone in the long run. Simply say: "I am on the most powerful food regimen on the planet and I am not allowed to eat sugar or refined carbohydrates". This might seem like a cold and disruptive answer, but it is your sincerity that will leave a lasting sense of respect and even admiration. Even if you just couldn't say no to that "Oh just this once", you can still address your concern for eating healthy food and motivate your aunt to give better choices for next time. You must be honest with yourself and with others. Surrounding yourself with people that care about their health as much as you do can be a challenge, but with consistent effort and discipline, people around you can also start to change. Be gentle, yet effective to handle any situation that causes your internal alarm to panic. Listen to yourself and take action to remain in *Pervasive Homeostasis*.

Acting on your *Identification locks* can be a problem for some people because they can make a person seem close-minded or panicky among what others see as harmless indulgence. But for a Delta-human, the *identification locks* are the miraculous work of your mind telling you what is good and bad for your survival.

POINT 3:

REASONS, CONCLUSIONS, EVIDENCE

America has for many years been labeled as the country of obese people. Currently, most Americans are so sick that every year more than 70% of them die prematurely from chronic disease. Nearly every single adult in our society is

classified as sick. So many citizens are sick that it is natural
for them to believe that getting sick is a natural sign of aging
and view their health problems as a badge of maturity rather
than of abnormal body functions caused by poor nutrition.
Most of these diseases are preventable just by changing our
diets. Carelessness in regards to food has taken away many
quality years from the lives of productive Americans, yet
other countries in Europe, for instance, are very aware of
these health issues and have responded by actively banning
substances like fluoride, BPA plastics, pesticides, hormones,
etc… Americans must begin catching up on the things that
matter regarding quality of life. America is special; it does
things a bit differently than most countries, in America,
people actually have to want the change and start buying
quality food when they can.

America is a country of marked individualism and freedom.
This is why we must partake into *principled eating* at an
individual level; The Delta-human System is here to support
the change. With principled eating, we can start to reverse
America's un-principled eating habits. By changing the way
we think about food, American consumers can radically
change the demand pattern. If we all demanded the best, we
would only produce the best in the first place. Instead of
spending so much of our land and resources in the production
of wheat and corn, we could be producing

healthier vegetables and could even spare much needed grass-lands for live-stock. This change must happen first at an individual level, with our children, where the notion of engaging in "sustainable organic farming" is acknowledged not as a "low-class and rudimentary practice", but as an "in-demand, rewarding and very noble enterprise". Once this becomes clear, then the spread from individuals to families and to community can follow. The goal is to attain previously un-thought of levels of well-being and prosperity by using knowledge, technology and teamwork in a heroic stance against trying to cheat nature. Delta-humans are effective pioneers of this change.

Taking a look at the rest of the American continent (central and south), we can see that our fellow men there are catching up fairly quick to the American influence. Mexico for instance, consumes more soda per person than any other country and is linked to an unprecedented number of diabetics. In contrast, Japan has addressed the problem by making available a commercial version of sodas with the natural sweetener stevia instead of sugar. They have been doing so for over 40 years now. Moreover, Argentina has switched to a less active and computerized work force in which they eat more and move less. Argentina has an obesity rate of 75% of the total population according to a 2010 report from the World Health Organization (WHO). If America is the economic model to follow, we are doing a very poor job at leading in other important areas, particularly health. We must emphasize on the prevention of disease and not on the cures, which are much harder to deal with. We can only do this by adopting *principled eating*.

Besides these ugly facts, do you happen to know a friend or relative with high cholesterol or diabetes? Or do you have a friend with acne problems consequence not of hormonal disorders, but of a diet rich in refined carbohydrates, highly processed dairy, and excessive sugar amounts? Do you know someone with low-energy levels? It is rare if your answer is no, but instead of focusing only on the causes for our problems, lets learn by **contrasts**; what does the **Delta-human (A)** do so differently from the **average-American (B)**?

A) The Delta man	B) The average American
A) The **Delta** man or woman drinks 6 to 8 glasses or more of pure water depending on the particular climate and activity level they are experiencing. They	B) The **average-American** will usually be in a state of chronic dehydration. When thirsty, he or she will consume liquids like sugary juices and

are not chronically dehydrated like the average American. They drink plain water, cleansing and renewing their bodily fluids, while stimulating the cleansing of all other organs in their bodies.	sodas. Also caffeinated beverages or alcohols which have diuretic /dehydrating effects on the body.
A) The **Delta-human** understands that mineral deficiencies should be prevented. They take mineral supplements to counteract the effects of our mineral-depleted farm lands and mineral-poor drinking water. *NOTE: A healthy way to get trace minerals is by using Sea, Celtic or Himalayan salts in your diet. Not refined table salt which has no trace elements worth ingesting. In regards to nutritional supplements, NEW CHAPTER ORGANICS brand of multivitamins are recommended for their certified organic and GMO	B) The **average-American** may be overweight, yet be anemic, mineral deficient, or malnourished. This can lead to a myriad of health complications, poor performance in school or work, and even premature aging due to poor nutrition. *NOTE: Minerals and trace elements are very important to the overall health of the body. In addition, just as magnesium and vitamin D are needed in the absorption of calcium, many other basic trace elements are needed for other bodily processes that are crucial for optimum

free sources, however, there are many other good ones out there for you to consider. (The Delta System has not been paid to promote any products, this is just an honest opinion).

health. There are many examples on how to restore the body's natural vitality by correcting mineral deficiencies. For more information on this topic, read "Colloidal Minerals and Trace Elements" by Marie-France Muller.

A)   The **Delta-human** commands a powerful system of food-group identification, its natural implications (proper food combining, timing, acid-alkaline properties of food, real foods, understands individual caloric needs, etc.), and is disciplined in applying his knowledge despite cultural, financial, or social pressures to eat otherwise.

B)   The **average-American** ignores or simply disregards the rules of food combining, individual caloric needs, alkalinity/acidity properties of food, often mixing all the possible food groups in one sitting and taking the bloating, irritability and poor digestion as something normal. Unfortunately, there are too many people living in a weakened state of chronic metabolic acidosis and other food-related problems today. Ironically, many Americans know about good food choices, yet they are not applying their knowledge

	because of cultural pressures or convenience.
A)　The **Delta-human** obeys natural digestive cycles. Eats during the 12 hour *energy production cycle* and rests from food for the following 12 hour *restorative cycle*.	B)　The **average-American** will eat at any time of the day and often eat heavily right before bed. Digestion is impaired, and the stomach is not given enough rest to work properly the next day.
A)　The **Delta-human** has less stress in life because of the control and discipline over food and consequently over life. He or she has sufficient rest and is able to accommodate a 25 minute nap during the day to refresh his attention span when needed and also takes time to exercise and stretch their bodies. The Delta-human procures good quality nutrients, and feels vibrant and more able to do his/her job at work or study in	B)　The **average-American** lives a stressful life with little or no control over his/her resources. This only gets worsened by the low-quality nutrition content of their food, poor digestion of it, and disregard for proper rest. Instead, he or she relies on energy boosters such as caffeine or "energy" drinks. These chemicals affect physical and mental well-being in an unnatural way. The average-American dreads going to work

41

school. A Delta-human improves the life of those around him by strengthening their self-control and being unaffected by external stimuli.

because he lives physically and mentally fatigued.

Note: Attention capacity is limited. Sleeping/napping recharges attention capacity. Many people go through life with total disregard for sleep. This is a main reason why people can't focus at work or find a class interesting in school. When tired, everything can seem blurry or irrelevant. This inability to use attention, blocks the ability to see continuity, making the subject seem boring.

POINT 4:

FOOD CLASSIFICATION SYSTEM

Humans are supposed to eat simple meals that our bodies can properly metabolize. The Delta-human (you) should get into an "eat-simple-routine" by understanding that cultural food usually mixes all food groups in one plate. This habitual mixing of food groups actually troubles digestion, produces gases, causes bloating and irritability in the stomach. In the long term, it may lead to ulcers and irritable bowel syndrome. Eating simple meals is "simply" better for you.

What evidence is there that we should eat simple? It is a matter of looking at our long line of evolution. Our hunter-gatherer ancestors ate one naturally occurring food at a time. For example, they would find a cherry tree and eat cherries until they were satisfied for the moment, then, later that day, they would hunt-down a wild boar and gorge on it. They did not mix all food groups in one plate as we do today. Our stomachs are just not used to this modern mixing trend. Some people tolerate this mixing more than others; however, if you are new to eating simple, do not be surprised when a feeling of crisp lightness follows after each time you apply *principled eating*.

The food pyramid commonly found in bread and cereal packages has been accepted and unquestioned by most Americans today. Don't fall for it without questioning it. It is simply not natural to rely mostly on grains and cereals. A diet based on cereals and grains is the same diet we give to our cattle to abnormally fatten them. Besides, we have the Paleo-diet argument that states that grains have to be cooked to be eaten, but since our evolutionary ancestors have eaten everything mostly raw for the past millions of years, and only dominated fire for the past four-hundred thousand years, then we can infer that we are not natural grain eaters, and since our genes are not accustomed to survive on mostly grains, then it does not make sense for grains to be identified as our primary food, and doing so, goes against historical human nature. It simply is not true that we can survive best on a diet based mostly on grains, and much less, refined grains. Another thing about the pyramid: food groups in the pyramid are not to be served all at the same time. There are feasible physiological reasons why we should have food combining rules. To ensure proper digestion, food groups should be eaten according to the rules of proper food combining. This is also the first step in getting rid of bloated stomachs. Many men and women (women especially) often complain from that hard-to-lose belly fat. Exercise alone will not flatten a belly that is bloated by gases produced by poor digestion. For details on how to get rid of this condition examine the rules and diagram that follows.

TYPES OF FOOD:

HIGH-STARCH CARBOHYDRATES: Cereals/Grains (rice, wheat, corn, oats, barley, etc.), avocado, carrots, eggplant, pasta, pumpkin, squash, radish, potatoes, yams, etc.

NON-STARCHY CARBOHYDRATES (high in water-content), lettuce, spinach, cress, arugula, broccoli, cabbage, cauliflower, celery, cucumber, green beans, kale, okra, cilantro, parsley, peppers, seaweed, etc..

FOODS HIGH IN PROTEIN: dairy, beans, chickpeas, lentils, chicken, beef, fish, nuts, seeds, etc.

FRUIT: apple, lemon, fig, pear, cherry, orange, mango, banana, etc.

3 Combination Rules

1) Proteins or carbohydrates:

<u>Avoid mixing proteins with starchy-carbohydrates.</u> Proteins require an acidic environment (hydrochloric acid) to digest. Proteins should be mixed only with vegetables that do not contain starch such as leafy greens (welcome lots of salads into your diet). High-starch carbohydrates require an alkaline environment to digest because of the enzymes required to break down starch; when mixed with protein, the acid and alkaline environments get disrupted (acid and alkaline cancel each other out), and the food sits in the stomach longer than it should while fermenting, releasing gases, and causing bloating. Hamburgers, sandwiches and pastas with meat, are all examples of heavy combinations that mix carbohydrates (bread and pastas) with protein. They may cause you to feel full for longer, but they will also burden proper digestion. This is why you should allow at least 3 hours between eating high-starch-carbohydrates meals and protein meals. Doing this allows you to better absorb the nutritional content of your food without digestive hindrance. Also, different types of protein such as seeds and nuts, need different acidic concentrations to digest than those of chicken or beef because of their chemical-fatty make-up and other enzymatic properties, so it is best not to mix these kinds of proteins.

2) Eat fruits alone

Fruits require very little digestion; mixing fruit with starches (pasta, rice) neutralizes the alkaline environment needed for the digestion of carbohydrates producing indigestion. Fruits mixed with proteins will neutralize the acidic environment required for protein digestion. Undigested proteins putrefy in bacterial decomposition and produce toxins. Allow at least an hour to digest the fruit before eating other food groups. After any meal, wait at least two hours to ingest fruit. Some fruits like berries and melons which are quick to ferment are especially best to be eaten alone. Slowly fermenting fruits such as apples, bananas and coconut, on the other hand, can be mixed with other foods with less discomfort.

3) <u>Forget about desserts and sugar</u>. Desserts usually consist of a vicious mixture of either sugar and refined carbohydrates (pastries), or processed sugary-dairy (ice cream and milk shakes). Use mental discipline (and your identification locks) to avoid desserts. In a restaurant, just pay the bill and go; you will feel better you did. At the supermarket, don't even go near the sweet isle.

RULES OF PROPER FOOD COMBINING

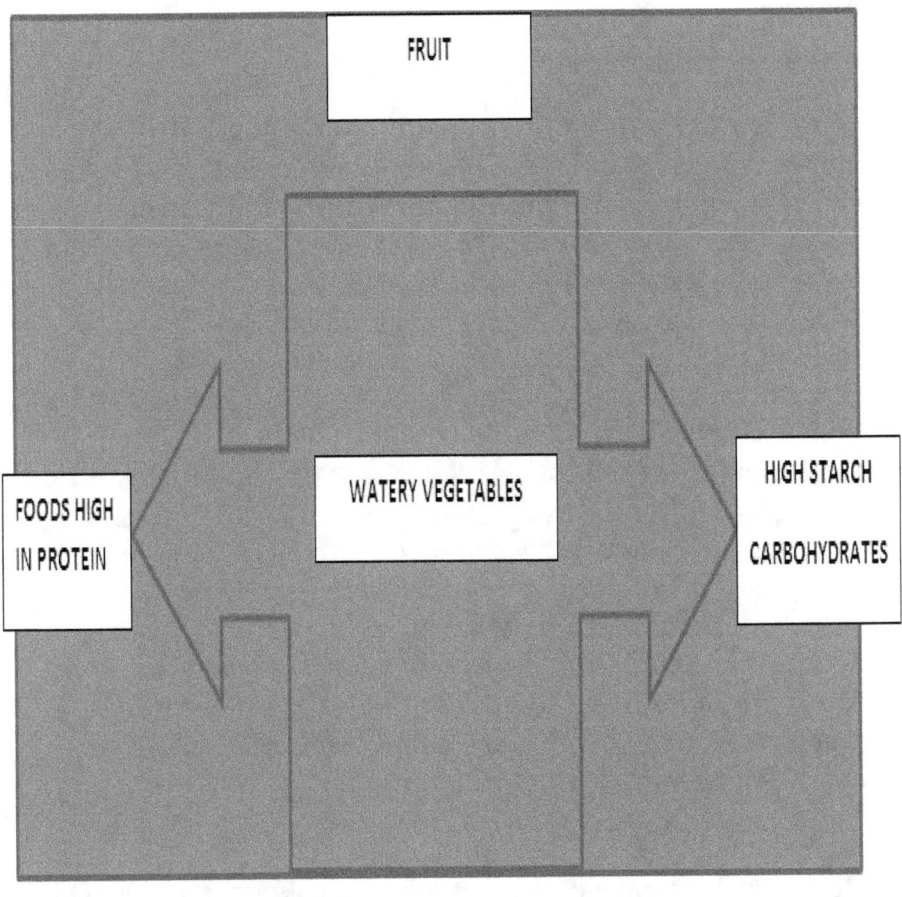

POINT 5:

DIGESTIVE CYCLES

There are 2 digestive cycles operating continuously in all human beings. They have a behavior similar to that of night and day; a period of about 12 hours from start to finish. The 12 hour day-time period is the *energy production cycle*. This is the time of the day where food is required for your body to generate energy. A Delta-human will program all his meals within this 12 hour time frame. For example, having breakfast at 7am and your last meal of the day preferably 30 minutes before 7pm, would be optimal. Having a 6pm last-meal usually works best, as it gives you time to eat slowly and digest before the cycle ends at 7pm. The 12-hour night-time-period that follows is the *restorative cycle* in which your body assimilates all the nutrients you gave it during the previous cycle. In the *restorative cycle*, your body needs nothing but water. If you have not been following your digestive cycles, you should start right away in order to realize a better digestion, less toxin retention, and a better overall health and energy.

Occasional skipping of meals such as breakfast (the easiest to skip) can be viewed as a form of *intermittent fasting*. It is a way of using energy in your body that has been stored as fat. This has many cleansing benefits that can help your body renew itself. While fasting, always remember to drink plenty of water to neutralize gastric juices. Always keep your body in check, the Delta-human System recommends no more than 3 skipped meals per week.

Another great practice is to take in the most energetic foods such as fruits, sprouted breads, avocados, oatmeal or raw vegetables in the morning to mid-afternoon and intake protein in the later part of the day. This is because the energy from fruits, carbohydrates and good fats (avocado, flax-seed oil, olive oil, etc.) are more readily available for energy production. Meat and other protein-rich foods on the other hand, are better eaten later in the day because proteins are the building blocks of muscle and tissue repair. This repair happens mostly while you sleep, so it is best to have most of your protein needs as your dinner and not breakfast. Another reason to eat your protein later in the day is that you can just sleep better. Meat will take a lot of digestive work to be metabolized and this makes a person feel tired right after eating it. Thus, eating a high protein meal around 6:30pm, assuming you will go to bed at 10pm, is a great way to promote good rest. Eating meat in the late afternoon is a very ancient practice. According to Joseph SB Morse, writer of the book "the evolution diet", our ancestors, the hunter-gatherers, used to go hunting and be compelled to eat massive amounts of meat after their mid-day hunting. They had to finish their prey; there were no refrigerators to keep the meat from going bad, so they ate most of it on the spot. It is probable that they would then take the leftovers back with them to their settlement to give to their families. Deserved periods of rest followed from their exhausting hunting expedition.

Digestion, Exercise and Stretching

For the best digestion to occur, you should exercise at least 20 minutes per day, 3-5 times per week. This must be a cardiovascular activity such as walking fast, jogging, running or other aerobic activities that get your blood pumping and your lungs breathing to capacity. Cardio-activity will also trigger a more powerful digestion, a more efficient elimination of toxins through sweat, and increased blood circulation and oxygenation of the brain and limbs. From exercise, the body experiences significant benefits including rejuvenation. Exercise is the real fountain of youth. Feel and look 10-15 years younger by implementing good exercise habits in your life. Memory and happiness are also boosted in the process. Your immune system is strengthened and the lungs are optimized. Weight-lifting is a great addition to aerobic exercise; however, it does not substitute for it. With weight-lifting, you build strength, but you do not get all the benefits of aerobic exercise. The other key ingredient is stretching. A person living in a state of limited motion can over time, become stiff and tense. Stretching is a great way to boost flexibility and feel great at any age. Daily stretching on just a simple carpet or rug, can greatly improve your well-being. Always remember to stretch before and after exercise.

Resting from exercise is encouraged for proper recovery from intense activity. The Delta System suggests to exercise aerobically 3-5 days per week, and thereby to rest for at least 2 days per week.

Napping

Every day-mid-day naps of about 25 minutes should be everyone's solution to recharging attention capacity naturally, instead of inducing it with caffeine or other "energy-boosters". Most people have the notion that naps are necessary only for toddlers. The truth is that naps are good for everyone. This fact should be recognized as integral to human nature and be considered as important as having a lunch break. A 25 minute mid-day nap should be standard for all the employees of an efficient business. Production would be renewed with intensity. Imagine focused workers instead of tired, grumpy and passive workers. Today however, this may sound impossible to accomplish because this need has not been given the importance it deserves, and many businesses do not have the willingness, the facilities or the knowledge to apply napping for employees, but when possible, get at least 25 minutes of rest around the time of the day when you would normally feel tired or unable to focus. There have been some interesting accounts from creative Delta-humans who work regular jobs, yet do clever things to get those 25 minutes of mental rest. You may share your personal experiences with this practice at deltahuman.com. Nap and feel your attention come back with renewed intensity.

POINT 6:

ACID/ALKALINE

In an alkaline state, the human body thrives. Besides dehydration, the average American is living in a state of chronic acidosis. In an acidic state, your body is more vulnerable to diseases such as arthritis, infections, and even cancer. Dr. George W. Crile, past head of the Crile Institute in Cleveland and one of the world's greatest surgeons says: "There is no natural death. All deaths from so called natural causes are merely the end-point of a progressive acid saturation." Most processed food products are acidifying, such as breakfast cereals, cheeses, pizzas, hamburgers, etc. You should identify acid yielding foods (See Acid-Alkaline chart) and try to avoid them at least 2- 3 times per week in what Delta-humans call *"**Alkaline days**"*. For more information on ***Alkaline days,*** please refer to the *"Sample diets"* section of the appendix to see a dietary example.

Realize how alkaline foods from the chart below are mostly fruits and vegetables that can be eaten *RAW*. Do you see the connection? The path to health includes large amounts of alkalizing vegetables, fruits, seeds, nuts and spices.

Recent studies have discovered that lowering homocysteine levels in the blood can significantly minimize the risk of cardiovascular diseases such as strokes. Leafy vegetables, almonds, bananas, sunflower seeds, and sprouted seeds, for instance, all contain the necessary B-vitamins to reduce homocysteine. These foods happen to be alkalizing foods. This means that by alkalizing your diet with foods rich in B-vitamins, you can also reduce homocysteine and acidity in the blood.

Meat, on the other hand, can be acidifying, and this is why it should not be eaten more than 5 times per week. Meat, however, is packed with essential nutrients that are hard to substitute. Eggs and organ meats like liver and kidney contain many essential B-vitamin co-factors that reduce homocysteine. White bread, doughnuts or cakes are also acidifying foods, yet we do not need them for their nutrient content at all, in fact we are better-off without them.

Eating animal protein is healthy and natural, but days in which we subsist only on alkaline fruits, vegetables, greens and a small amount of nuts (a handful), give the body a chance to be in a healing alkaline state, without acidity disrupting the healing environment.

 Alkaline days and occasional *intermittent fasting* (with sufficient pure water) are also extremely good for detoxifying your metabolism. This is the way one rests from over-eating in a similar way to how we rest from intense exercise. Clearer, more beautiful skin is also achieved this way. The most beautiful skin is that of an alkaline-balanced person that also avoids sugar, refined carbohydrates, hydrogenated oils and other refined ingredients, but that intakes an appropriate amount of EFA's (Essential Fatty Acids) like the ones found in olive oil and salmon, for a healthy skin from the inside out.

FOOD CATEGORY	High Alkaline	Alkaline	Low Alkaline
BEANS, VEGETABLES, LEGUMES	Vegetable Juices, Parsley, Raw Spinach, Broccoli, Celery, Garlic, Barley Grass	Carrots, Green Beans, Lima Beans, Beets, Lettuce, Zucchini, Carob	Squash, Asparagus, Rhubarb, Fresh Corn, Mushrooms, Onions, Cabbage, Peas, Cauliflower, Turnip, Beetroot, Potato, Olives, Soybeans, Tofu
FRUIT	Dried Figs, Raisins	Dates, Blackcurrant, Grapes, Papaya, Kiwi, Berries, Apples, Pears	Coconut, Sour Cherries, Tomatos, Oranges, Cherries, Pineapple, Peaches, Avocados, Grapefruit, Mangoes, Strawberries, Papayas, Lemons, Watermelon, Limes
GRAINS, CEREALS			Amaranth, Lentils, Sweetcorn, Wild Rice, Quinoa, Millet, Buckwheat

56

FOOD CATEGORY	Low Acid	Acid	High Acid
BEANS, VEGETABLES, LEGUMES	Sweet Potato, Cooked Spinach, Kidney Beans	Pinto Beans, Navy Beans	Pickled Vegetables
FRUIT	Blueberries, Cranberries, Bananas, Plums, Processed Fruit Juices	Canned Fruit	
GRAINS, CEREALS	Rye Bread, Whole Grain Bread, Oats, Brown Rice	White Rice, White Bread, Pastries, Biscuits, Pasta	

POINT 7:

CONCLUSION

Briefly stated:

1)   Food is for energy to survive, not for enjoyment. Again, the person seeking enjoyment as the primary motive for eating, will undoubtedly succumb to the sweet or salty garbage that are compulsively competing for the attention of that person's palate.

2)   Respect the Food combination rules by remembering that foods are divided into 4 groups; fruits, proteins, watery vegetables, and starchy carbohydrates, which should be consumed according to the 3 rules of food combining.

3)   Be aware of alkaline and acid producing foods to ensure a larger amount of alkaline foods and prevent chronic acidosis.

4)   Eliminate sugar and sugary foods from your diet. Identify the foods and drinks that only "appear to be healthy" but that have high sugar/fructose content or that are highly processed or refined. Check all ingredients.

5)   Understand the importance of staying hydrated. You should take around 3 quarts to a gallon of water per day depending on your activity levels and climate. Try to take 1-2

glasses of water 30 minutes before meals and when thirsty.
NOTE: Large amounts of water are recommended for people
in the process of change from conventional eating to
principled eating in order to detoxify themselves and prepare
their bodies for a more pure and natural nutrition. Once you
adopt the Delta-human System's way to *principled eating*,
you will need somewhat less water, (5-8 glasses per day)
since there is less acid and toxic build-up.

6)   Get *real foods* to the best of your ability and try to get
them from natural/organic sources.

7)   Respect your digestive cycles by eating within the
energy-production cycle and resting from food in the
restorative cycle.

8)   Know your body's caloric needs. How much is enough?
Do you feel that you are eating too much or too little?
Compare it and adapt to your unique needs. Take in quality
calories from a variety of quality food.

9)   Master the principles shown and apply them every day
with   △   as the point of reference to everything else. This
requires independent thought. Act on your *Identification
locks* with prior planning and some research. When in social
situations, use honesty and gentleness to protect yourself
from disrupting pressure. Lead others by example.

Here we can see the *Homeostasis Octagon,* the diagram that reminds you about important factors needed to achieve your own personal homeostasis.

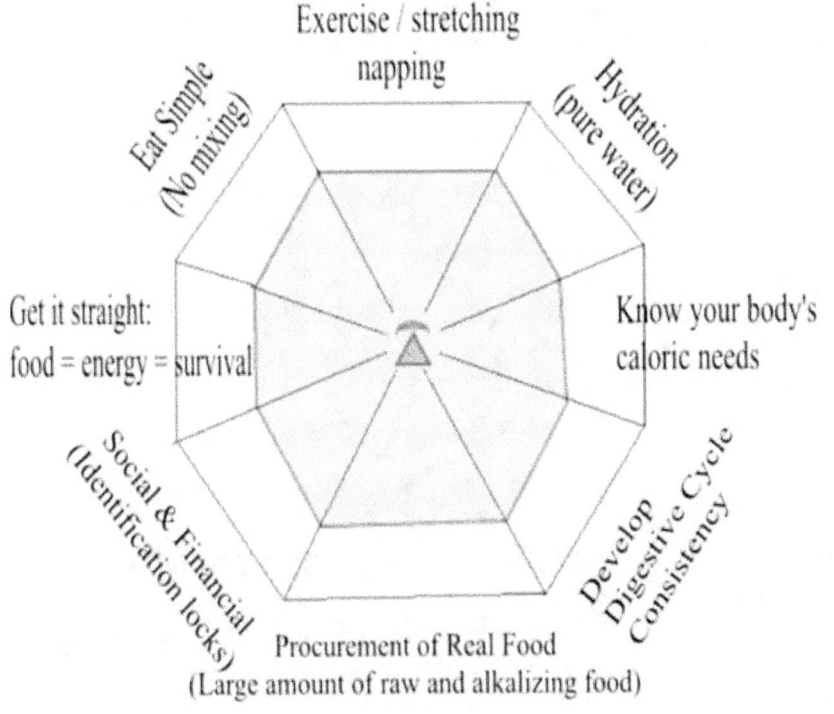

Exercise / stretching napping

Hydration (pure water)

Eat Simple (No mixing)

Get it straight: food = energy = survival

Know your body's caloric needs

Social & Financial (Identification locks)

Develop Digestive Cycle Consistency

Procurement of Real Food
(Large amount of raw and alkalizing food)

NOTE:

It is important to understand the previous diagram for the
following passage to have force. Test your knowledge by
reading the 9 points in the conclusion and analyzing the
homeostasis octagon's factors in detail. If any one point is
not clear, re-read the section on that topic and continue until
clear.

READ THE FOLLOWING PASAGE OUT LOUD WHEN
READY*

61

In the past, I have succumbed to failure with food, but today it
is different, for today I am a new being that begets health and
new knowledge. It is my inner-most duty to give my body a
complete nutrition that satisfies it's energy and nutrient needs.
This is more fundamental and basic to accomplish than other
immediate goals in life because great food choices improve my
mental and physical performance, thus improving my chances
to attain those other goals. I am now activated to procure the
best food for myself by applying these powerful principles to
my food choices. I am removing any negative habits that I do
not want in my life. I am walking my natural path and my
habits must be aligned with it. I am striving for beauty and
health. I am willing to invest in my ideal state of homeostasis.
I consciously monitor and adjust the quality and quantity of all
food according to what feels best and is best for my body in the
long term. I am now more able to establish my personal
homeostasis. I re-enforce this winning mentality with every
day that I read this passage. Every day, from now on, through
the months and years to come, I will have more control over
the important aspects of food. I am excited to get to know how
controlling my food can improve my body and also the bodies
of people I care about. This is the most important journey of
my life. This is my journey towards taking responsibility for
my health. I am hereby on my way to become a human with
higher consciousness, improved mental and physical abilities,
natural physical beauty, and a greater appreciation for life...
A Delta-human; a stable human.

Always in homeostasis.

The Value of Independence

For a Delta-human, independence is one of the most highly regarded values. By being independent, it means that you have broken your dependency to anyone or anything. The key to unlock your independence lies within you through the grasping of the appropriate knowledge, and outside of you, in your relationships to other people (their influence over you), the control of your own unfounded impulses, and the control of your own resources (financial and spatial).

When you grasp the appropriate knowledge, you become actively engaged in looking for inconsistencies. When new knowledge comes into you awareness, your mind instantly starts differentiating according to your notions of good and bad. You might shockingly come to realize that you are now over-reacting to food after absorbing this knowledge (*Identification locks*). As you go through the pages of the Delta System, your mind begins giving you warnings every time there is danger of breaking your homeostasis; your metabolic balance. This break in homeostasis might be happening to you every day right now, and for all you know, this is normal. In reality, it is neither normal nor desirable to remain ignorant of your ideal state. The right knowledge is necessary to be able to identify what is wrong with the way we think about food. Initial over-reacting is normal, and with time (months to years) you will be able to adjust your needs according to your own requirements for *homeostasis.*

Financial resources are an important part for anyone applying the Delta-human System. If you have control over your budget, then you can consider allocating higher resources to your food selections. You will want to invest in higher quality food (explained in the Delta-human System) and not think of it as a loss but as an absolute gain, an investment for greater mental and physical performance.

An individual that has no control over basic resources such as, living space, food, or money, is an individual who is probably not really acting on his/her own conclusions. This individual might suffer from depression or a sense of impotency and disorder. To get things right, you have to worry about your finances and your habits. You must take full responsibility for your environment as you are the one operating in it. To have the privilege to act on your own conclusions, you must exert the hard mental and physical effort required to love yourself and to love others. If you have the will to succeed and help humanity advance, you are going to want to live like a Delta-human.

64

APPENDIX

The Glycemic index below is a useful resource in comparing and contrasting types of foods that quickly affect the blood-sugar levels. You want to pick foods with low-glycemic indexes because they are slowly metabolized and give out a more steady supply of energy throughout the day. Low-glycemic foods help keep your blood-sugar levels normal by not triggering abnormal insulin reactions. This is why cakes and doughnuts, for instance (high-glycemic foods), give you sudden energy spikes followed by fatigue or sugar crashes.

NOTE: High glycemic vegetables like carrots, parsnips and beats, are not unhealthy despite their high-glycemic loads. It would be beneficial, however; to eat them with another carbohydrate such as avocado, since they are all starchy carbohydrates, you are not mixing food groups, and the healthy fats from the avocado, will buffer the sugar spike and normalize the absorption of high-glycemic energy.

Glycemic Indexes of Common Foods

All values are aprox. and may vary from other sources.

Breads & Grains		Boxed Cereals	
Bagel	72	Bran based cereal	49
Baguette, French	95	Corn cereal	74
Barley	25	Granola cereal	83
Bread, whole wheat	73	Muesli	54
Bulgar	46	Oat cereal	66
Cornmeal	68	Rice cereal	89
Croissant	67	Shredded wheat cereal	67
Dark rye	76		
Doughnut	76	Legumes	
Hamburger bun	61	Baked beans	40
Millet	71	Black beans (boiled)	30
Oatmeal (old-fashioned	48	Garbanzos (boiled)	34
Rice, brown	55	Kidney beans	23
Rice, white	56	Kidney beans (canned)	52
Spaghetti, white	41	Lentils	28
Spaghetti, whole wheat	32	Lima beans (boiled)	32
Tortilla (corn)	52	Pinto beans (boiled)	38
Waffle	76	Soy beans	15
Wheat kernels	48		

66

Dairy		Fruits		Beverages	
Ice cream, vanilla	60	Apple	40	Apple juice	40
Skim milk	32	Apricots	57	Chocolate milk	33
Whole milk	25	Banana	51	Cola soda	75
Yogurt, plain	14	Cantaloupe	65	Fruit punch	67
Yogurt, w/fruit	36	Cherries	22	Sports drink	78
		Dates	103	Lemonade, sweetened	54
		Grapes	43	Orange juice	50
		Kiwi	52	Pineapple juice	46
Starchy Vegetables		Orange	48	Soft drinks	63
Carrots (boiled)	49	Papaya	58	Tomato juice	38
Carrots (raw)	92	Peach	42		
French fries	75	Pear	33		
Parsnips (boiled)	97	Pineapple	66		
Potatoes, new (baked)	59	Prunes	15		
Potatoes, red (boiled)	93	Raisins	64		
Potatoes, sweet (baked	52	Watermelon	72		
Potatoes, white, mash	70				
Yam (baked)	54				

67

Delta-Human List of Recommended Foods

Color	Warning	
Grey =	In moderate amounts	
FRUITS	**LEAFY VEGETABLES**	spinach
apples	alfalfa	swiss chard
avocado	arugula	**VEGETABLES**
bananas	bok choy	carrots
blueberries	broccoli	cucumber
cantaloupe	cabbage	garlic
cherries	celery	mushrooms
figs	collard	onion
guava	cress	parsnips
kiwi	kale	rutabagas
lemon	kelp	squash
lime	lettuce	turnips
oranges	mustard cress	yams
pineapple	nopal	zucchini
prickly pear	parsnip greens	**SPICES**
raspberries	purslane	basil
tomatillo	sea weed	cayenne pepper

	ANIMAL FOOD	LEGUMES
celtic salt		
cinnamon	beef: free range, grass-fed	green beans
clover	buffalo: free range, grass-fed	sprouted mung beans
ginger	dairy: raw, grass-fed	**WHOLE GRAINS**
himalayan salt	edible insects	barley
mustard	eggs: free range, organic	brown rice
nutmeg	fish: low mercury/PCB's	old fashioned oats
paprika	naturally raised chicken	**SEEDS/ NUTS**
pepper	naturally raised goat	almonds
sea salt	naturally raised lamb	chia
stevia	naturally raised turkey	coconut
turmeric	ostrich	flax
OILS	pork, organic	hazelnuts
avocado	rabbit	sprouted alfalfa
coconut	raw honey	sprouted quinoa
olive		walnuts

SAMPLE DIETS:

NOTE: Following the dietary principles outlined in the Delta-human System takes time and a strong determination. The Delta-human System is well worth the extra effort because once these principles are adopted and sustained for about a month, you will automatically apply them at home without much effort thereafter. You will be living, working, studying, etc., yet at the same time, be getting all the benefits and incalculable advantages of flawless digestion. Sometimes breaking the rules will seem impossible because we get involved with undisciplined people and social events. This is the biggest challenge for most Delta-humans. It is in social situations in which we seem to have no control, where we should look to regain the discipline with self-assertion and strength of character. Remember that all the good food choices you make really add-up. The more you last on a great food regimen, the more you will want to stay that way because of the realized benefits. Get into a state of sustained focus when confronted with social pressure and always try to remain honest and follow the food choices that <u>you</u> agree on. Always have a plan, a list, or a reminder of what your food plan is for that day.

The Following 4 diets are precise principled samples, not "fancy recipes". Observe the rules they adhere to. By understanding food combining, digestive cycles, acid/alkaline properties of food, hydration, exercise, and caloric needs, you will be able to customize your own diet to meet your personal likes and needs. Meanwhile, you are encouraged to follow these simple "on-the-go" samples using real foods:

How to follow the sample diets:

In a week: Alternate Diets 1,2 &3. Include a pair of

Alkaline days (Diet 4). For example:

Sun - 4/ Mon – 1/ Tue – 2 / Wed – 4 / Thu – 3 / Fri – 1 / Sat – 2

SAMPLE DIET #1 *(Target: 2,400 calories, protein-30%, fat-25%, carbs-40%, naturally occurring fructose from fruit -10%) See table below for Nutritional Details on Diet #1*

7:30 am 5 figs

8:00 am Aerobic Exercise (Running, jogging or fast walking)
- for 30 min.; always stretch before and after exercise

8:30 am Water

9:00 am 1 cup of old fashioned oatmeal with ground
- cinnamon and sea salt. A side of mashed avocado
- eaten with sliced carrots and celery sticks

11:00am Water

12:30pm 3 Scrambled eggs over baby spinach or spring mix
- salad (Pre-packaged organic salads are a good choice
- for convenience), garnished with fresh cilantro. Cook
- with 1 TBSP of coconut oil on a pan. No over-cooking

2:30 pm Fresh berries

3:30 pm Lightly steamed broccoli (2 cups) sprinkled with 1
- TBSP of freshly ground flax seeds. A side of baked yams
- with a dash of cinnamon

6:30 pm 8 oz. (grass-fed) steak, medium-rare, (boiled)
- with onions. Lettuce salad with 3 TBS of olive oil,
- season with a small pinch of Celtic Salt

7:30 pm Water only from now on

Caloric Breakdown of Diet #1 (This is just an example of the caloric and macronutrient breakdown of diet #1 for illustrative purposes. You do not have to do this every time you make a diet for yourself. This is, however; just one possible way to ensure your diet falls within ideal ratios.)

Item	Amount	Measurement	Protein (g)	Fat (g)	Natural Fructose (g)	Carbohydrates (g)	Total Calories
<Diet #1>							
Steak, brisket	8	oz	98.73	24			639
Avocado, hass	1	units	2	15		9	180
Figs (small)	5	units	1.5	0.65	40		210
Fresh berries	0.5	cups	0.54	0.24	10		42
Coconut oil	1	tbsp		13.03			117
Eggs, large	3	units	12.9	5.5		7.4	141
Cilantro	1	oz				1	0
Broccoli	2	cups	8.8	0.22		15	82
Oatmeal	1	cups	9	2.08		58.8	266
Flax seeds	2	tbsp	4.7	8.18		8.24	118.2
Olive oil	3	tbsp		39.81			358.2
Celery sticks (4" long)	3	units	0.09	0.01		0.36	0.48
Yam (baked)	1.5	cup	3.045	0.3		56.265	236.7
Carrot, raw	3	unit	2.04	0.54		20.7	88.5
TOTAL (g) >	SUM >	479.67	143.345	109.56	50	176.765	2479.08
		Actual Ratios	30%	23%	10%	37%	
Caloric Goal: 2300-2600		Ideal Ratios	22%	30%	13%	35%	

NOTE: Diet #1 is high in protein. Ideal ratios are the overall goal for the entire week, thus they balance out with the other daily diets.

By using an "on-the go" index card like the one below, anyone
can easily remember and keep track of the eating patterns
he/she must follow for that day. This is Diet #1 made simple.
Its divided in 4 quadrants which make it easier to divide the
hours of the day. Quadrant 1 is when rising, quadrant 2 is mid-
day, 3 is afternoon, and 4 is the remaining hours before going
to sleep.

Carry an index card like the one above for the specific diet you
are following for the day.

SAMPLE DIET # 2 (Tip: set your own desired target calories)

7:00 am An Orange
7:20 am Aerobic Exercise (Running, jogging or fast walking)
-      for 30 minutes (Exercise at your convenience, at any time
-      of the day)
7:50 am Water
8:20 am Alfalfa sprouts and soaked almonds (see pg. 20 for
-      instructions on how to soak almonds).
11:00am Water
11:30am Bowl of brown rice with lightly sautéed
-      broccoli and mushrooms using coconut oil.
1:00 pm Water 1-2 glasses of pineapple/ water blend,
-      no added sugar
2:30 pm Steamed zucchini, broccoli, mushrooms and
-      cauliflower mix w/ a sugarless dip of your choice.
4:30 pm Chicken breast over spinach and parsley salad
6:30 pm Boiled chicken thighs with crushed garlic, oregano,
-      and sliced onions
7:30 pm Only Water from now on

SAMPLE DIET # 3 (Tip: Try to incorporate a mid-day 25-min-nap every day)

7:30 am Grapefruit
8:00 am Aerobic Exercise (Running, jogging or fast walking)
-     for 30 minutes. Stretch all muscles first)
8:30 am Water
9:00 am Guacamole(Hass Avocado, jalapeno, red onion,
-     cilantro and Celtic salt) eat with brown rice or on
-     sprouted grain toast
11:00am Water
12:00pm Boiled (organic, grass-fed) calf liver (with your
-     choice of spices) over Arugula salad
2:00 pm Strawberries
3:00 pm Salad of raw vegetables (e.g.; carrot, lettuce,
-     avocado, cucumber, cauliflower, broccoli, parsley, and
-     olive oil with a pinch of sea salt)
6:30 pm Alaskan salmon steak (cooked medium) with
-     onions and peppers
8:30 pm Water Only from now on

Alkaline DAY #4 (2-3 times per week) On this day, avoid most acid producing foods. You can also use this light diet as an intermittent fasting day by skipping breakfast. Do drink plenty of water to dilute gastric juices when attempting any type of fasting.

7:30 am Pineapple
8:30 am Celery and baby carrot snack dipped in mashed
-        Hass avocado
9:00 am Alfalfa water-blend
10:00am Tea (lemon, decaf-green tea, peppermint,
-        or chamomile, etc.)
11:30am Steamed Kale with brussel sprouts, parsnips,
-        cabbage, mushrooms, crushed flax seeds, crushed
-        almonds, and olive oil/vinegar dressing
2:00 pm Cantaloupe
2:30 pm Water
3:00 pm Large raw vegetable salad (lettuce, cucumber,
-        seaweed, sprouted quinoa seeds, cauliflower, cilantro,
-        string beans, a pinch of sea salt
-        (You may add eggs or fish to this salad if you desire
-        additional protein)
6:30 pm, 1 ½ TBSP of Chia seeds
8:30 pm Water only from now on

5 IMPORTANT HINTS FOR SUCCESSFUL DIETING:

1. Get the food you will need for the week **in advance.**

2. Make *principled eating* a habit. This might seem too demanding, but in reality, it is the most time-saving and effective way to use this System.

3. Schedule your shopping trips on a planner or calendar, and write down the list of specific food items you will need for each day. This just works much better than trying to get all the ingredients when you are already at the supermarket. Besides, you can completely block the temptation to get the wrong foods if they are not on your shopping list. You won't need anything else...

4. Every night, work out the details of what you need to do in order to successfully implement the diet for the next day on a "3 x 5 index card" (See index card under Diet #1). If you are working, then you will have to arrange and pack everything in the morning. You must have proper food containers and a bag or backpack to fill each morning. You must eat according to the assigned times for each food.

5. Get rid of the sugary snacks and refined garbage lying around your house or office. It shouldn't be there in the first place.

Extra Tips:

1. To lose weight, reduce your intake of carbohydrates such as white bread, pasta, potatoes, rice, and corn (totally eliminate sugar and fructose syrups; the purest form of carbohydrates, this goes for everybody, not just those trying to get slim) because they are the main cause of insulin reactions that spike up the blood-sugar levels. Due to their processed nature and high-glycemic indexes, these carbohydrates and starches, trigger fat cells to grow. Particularly offensive, are cookies and pastries because they combine sugars with refined carbohydrates, burnt oils, and heavy dairy ' creams (A terrible mix of all food groups worsened by the preservatives necessary to keep them on the shelves.) If you want a healthy carb-load of cereal, old fashioned oatmeal is most recommended because it has glycemic levels below 60 and because rolled oats can be eaten uncooked as in the Swiss "muesli" cereal, which traditionally, adds fruit. The fruit however, should be eaten 30 minutes before the oatmeal for digestive purposes as described in the food combination rules. The glycemic index of the food you intake should be low because a low-glycemic index means that the energy of that food is absorbed slowly, and thus, is better metabolized. In fact, most refined or processed foods have high-glycemic indexes, so check the glycemic index chart in the appendix.

2. Protein: To maintain muscle mass, one should eat a gram of protein for every pound you weigh. For example, if you weigh 175 pounds, you should eat around 175 grams a day of protein. To increase muscle mass, one should eat 2 grams of protein per day for every pound you weigh. So if you weigh 175 pounds, you should take 350 grams of protein. (Heavy protein consumption should be accompanied by a heavy exercise routine, with 2-5 Cardiovascular and isometrics sessions of intense muscle building effort per week). Also include healthy fats in your diet to help in the absorption of the protein and to avoid protein poisoning also known as "rabbit starvation".

3. For those of you looking to gain healthy weight and muscle mass, protein alone will not do the trick. You will need carbs, greens, and fats to get enough calories in first. Failure to do so will make your body take the calories it needs from your starved muscles. The protein you ingest will instead be used to get energy and not to build muscle, so make sure you determine the amount of calories you need. (You can use the resources given in point 2: *"How much should we eat?"*) It is very

important for slim people trying to gain weight that they do indeed check how many calories they are consuming per day, and what their requirements are for their ideal weight. It is imperative that they not go looking for calories while ignoring the quality of the food they ingest to get them. It is not easy to select high calorie "real foods". A good choice again, is oatmeal, avocados, olive oil, and occasionally brown rice or sprouted grain breads.

4. About salts: Consume quality salts such as Sea, Celtic or Himalayan Salts to prevent the sodium deficiency known as Hyponatremia. Salt is lost in our sweat and perspiration. We are also at risk of losing salt if we drink too much distilled or heavily filtered water with no naturally occurring minerals. We do need to replace this salt sometimes, otherwise we may suffer from a sodium/potassium charge imbalance in our nervous system's impulses; this is characterized by a feeling of weakness, fatigue, headaches, and other symptoms. The recommendation for sodium limits in the Dietary Guidelines for Americans from the U.S. Department of Health and Human Services as well as the American Heart Association is 2,400 milligrams (mg) daily for adults. This is about the amount in 1 teaspoon of salt (2,300 mg). Normal sodium balance can be maintained

with 500 mg daily (or a little more than ¼ of a teaspoon of salt) NOTE: For people with high-blood pressure, consult your doctor first to see if this suggestion is right for you. This is not a substitute for medical advice. Especially for patients with serious illness or on medication.

5. Portion control is encouraged; eat portions that are about the size of your fist. Eating nutrient dense foods and healthy oils such as olive oil, will make you feel fuller and satisfied for a longer time, thus reducing the amount of food you crave for.

6. Digestion can be impaired by many factors, especially when we mix too many food groups or when we eat processed foods that contain no enzymes. You may want to consider the occasional use of digestive enzymes for times when you over-eat.

FINAL NOTES

The Delta-human system supports the notion that human beings are primarily carnivores with an organism to metabolize proteins, fats, and oils as explained by Dr. Robert Atkins in his bestselling diet books. This low-carbohydrate diet has been scientifically and experimentally confirmed. For more detailed information, see the *Atkins diet*, or the *Paleo diet* which also reaffirms the importance of protein-based diets. For those that opt to be vegetarian, they must find the proper protein balance within their food choices, but this book will not cover the vegan topic nor expand on its technicalities.

Do not eat meat that is burnt or charred to avoid consuming carcinogen chemicals known as HCA's. Also try to get meat from a good source, that is, cattle fed with grass or alfalfa, not grains. Look for livestock not injected with hormones or antibiotics, and that comes from an uncontaminated area to avoid dioxins. To ensure good meat, we should support and buy from local farmers that raise animals with knowledge about their nature and care.

Exercise, alkaline days, and proper rest, are necessary factors in your weekly routine. By getting these 3 things, you can better counteract the acidic reactions of eating meat and grains. We all have different levels of tolerance to certain foods, but most people can tolerate meat. Meat is very healthy and has been part of the human diet for thousands or even millions of years. Our intake of meat, however; has always been part of a nomadic and active lifestyle, do not fall into the sedentary trap; you must exercise regularly!

*Be sure to visit www.deltahuman.com/products.html for updates and offers.

As a Delta-human you take the
responsibility...

Maintain your well-being by procuring good
food and maintaining good eating habits. Do
so by applying these techniques to your life
with discipline.

First help yourself; get it right, feel good...
then you may better help others.

85

About the Author

Marcel Ostrow is one truly concerned citizen. He has exhibited a profound and un-canny interest in natural nutrition ever since he realized how controlling his dietary habits was the key to drastically improving his life in important ways. Throughout his college years and beyond, he had not engaged it fully, yet he knew something was wrong with the way most Americans thought and acted on their food choices. He became a Certified Sports Nutritionist by the American Sports & Fitness Association (ASFA), and has since, dedicated vast amounts of his time and resources to studying and applying natural nutrition principles to better his own life and that of the people willing to make a change in their life, particularly with food.

REFERENCES:

BOOKS

Holford, Patrick. *The New Optimum Nutrition Bible: Revised and Updated.* Crown Publishing Group, New York. 2004

Michalik, Steve. *Atomic Fitness: The alternative to drugs, steroids, wacky diets and everything else that's failed.* Laguna Beach, CA. Basic Health Publications, Inc. 2006

Muller, Marie-France, M.D.,N.D..PH.D.*Colloidal Minerals and Trace Elements: How to Restore the Body's Natural Vitality. Bernex, France. Healing Arts Press. 2005*

Cordain, Loren And Joe Frie. The Paleo Diet for Athletes: A Nutritional Formula for Peak Athletic Performance.USA, Rodale, Inc. 2005

Wharton, Charles Heizer, Ph.D. *Ten thousand years from Eden. Orlando, Fl. WinMark Publishing. 2001*

Morse, Joseph SB,*The Evolution Diet: What and how we were designed to eat.* San diego, Ca. Amelior Publishing Company, 2008

Anderson Bob. *Stretching: 30th anniversary edition,* Bolinas, Ca. Shelter Pub .Inc 2010

Menzer, Peter & D'aluisio Faith. *Man Eating Bugs: The art and science of eating insects.* Ten Speed Press, Material World Books .1998

87

INTERNET SOURCES AND ARTICLES

Slanker Ted, "GI and Omega 3 Nutritional Food Data" April 4th, 2010; October 31, 2010
http://www.texasgrassfedbeef.com/gi and omega 3 nutritional food data.htm#caution data is not always accurate

Harvard Business School of Public Health, Food Pyramids: what should you really eat? 2010
http://www.hsph.harvard.edu/nutritionsource/what-should-you-eat/pyramid/

According to Professor Melinda M. Manore of Oregon State University's Department of Nutrition and Exercise Sciences, http://www.supplementschat.org/homocysteine-b-vitamins-and-heart-disease.html

Dr. Ben Balzer's Paleolithic Diet Weblog 2010
http://paleolithicdiet.wordpress.com/2008/06/22/original-introduction/

Wholefoods: Unacceptable ingredients in food, 2010
http://www.wholefoodsmarket.com/products/unacceptable-ingredients.php

Eat Wild, the #1 source for grass-fed beef and facts, 2010
http://www.eatwild.com/healthbenefits.htm

National Cancer Institute: Heterocyclic Amines in Cooked Meat, 1994
http://www.cancer.gov/cancertopics/factsheet/Risk/heterocyclic-amines.

2010USDA Nutrient Database for Standard Reference, Release 14. US Department of Agriculture.Landers,

Daniel M. Landers *The influence of exercise on mental health, 2010* http://www.fitness.gov/mentalhealth.htm

Balancing Acid/Alkaline Foods: Foods http://www.trans4mind.com/nutrition/pH.html

Alkaline Food Chart: http://www.balance-ph-diet.com/acid_alkaline_food_chart.html

Environmental Defense Fund on Fish Safety: http://www.edf.org/page.cfm?tagID=17694..

Glycemic Index: Diabetesnet.com http://www.diabetesnet.com/diabetes_food_diet/glycemic_index.php#a xzz0yOIz5UVb

Campbell, Jonathan. What is Dioxin? http://www.cqs.com/edioxin.htm

Cynthia Kenyon, Jean Chang, Erin Gensch , Adam Rudner and Ramon Tabtiang A *C. elegans* mutant that lives twice as long as wild type. *Nature* 366(6454), 461-464 (1993) http://kenyonlab.ucsf.edu/Kenyon_et_al_Nature.pdf

Sang Whang, Acidosis Quotations from the "The Bob Livingston Letter", 2001 http://www.phbodybalance.com/acidosis.html

Please submit feedback, questions and comments to:
M@Deltahuman.com, you may also do so at
www.deltahuman.com

Serial No.

2X47Y-2QRZ5-8N18G-P41B3

www.ingramcontent.com/pod-product-compliance
Lightning Source LLC
Chambersburg PA
CBHW062049280526
45788CB00003B/1160